CW00525275

Keto Slow Cooker Ideas

50+ Keto Friendly And Easy Recipes For Your Slow Cooker

Elena Johnson

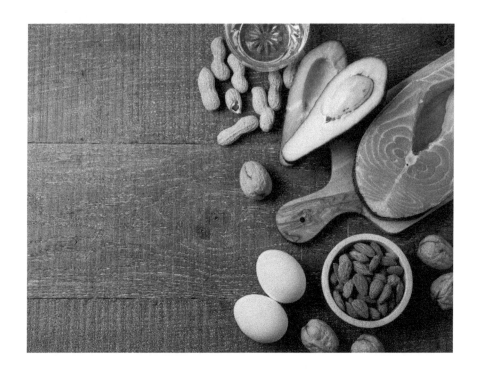

TABLE OF CONTENTS

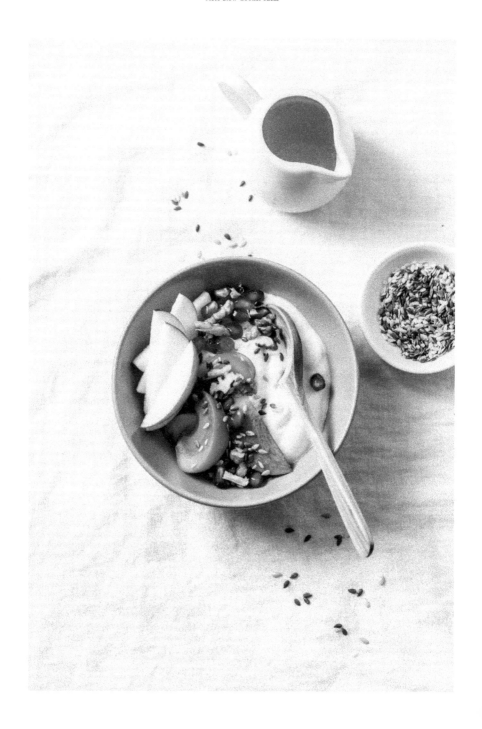

INTRODUCTION

The ketogenic diet is trendy, and for an excellent reason. It truly teaches healthy eating without forcing anyone into at risk. The success rate of keto is relatively high. While there are no specific numbers to suggest the exact rate, it is only fair to state that those who have the will to change their lifestyle and are okay adjusting to new eating habits, almost every one of them will make it through as a success story.

A diet that results in the production of ketone bodies by the liver is called a ketogenic diet; it causes your system to use fat instead of carbohydrates for energy. Limit your carbohydrate intake to a low level, causing some reactions. However, it is not a high protein diet. It involves moderate protein, low carbohydrate intake, and high fat intake.

Regardless of your lifestyle, everyone benefits from the keto diet in the following ways:

Weight Loss

Far more important than the visual aspect of excess weight is its negative influence on your body. Too much weight affects the efficiency of your body's blood flow, which in turn also affects how much oxygen your heart is able to pump to every part of your system. Too much weight also means that there are layers of fat covering your internal organs, which prevents them from working efficiently. It makes it hard to walk because it puts great pressure on your joints, and makes it very difficult to complete even regular daily tasks. A healthy weight allows your body to move freely and your entire internal system to work at its optimal levels.

Cognitive Focus

In order for your brain to function at its best, it needs to have balanced levels of all nutrients and molecules, because a balance allows it to focus on other things, such as working, studying, or creativity. If you eat carbs, the sudden insulin spike that comes with them will force your brain to stop whatever it was doing and to turn its focus on the correct breakdown of glucose molecules. This is why people often feel sleepy and with a foggy mind after high-carb meals. The keto diet keeps the balance strong, so that your brain does not have to deal with any sudden surprises.

Blood Sugar Control

If you already have diabetes, or are prone to it, then controlling your blood sugar is obviously of the utmost importance. However, even if you are not battling a type of diabetes at the moment, that doesn't mean that you are not in danger of developing it in the future. Most people forget that insulin is a finite resource in your body. You are given a certain amount of it, and it is gradually used up throughout your life. The more often you eat carbs, the more often your body needs to use insulin to break down the glucose; and when it reaches critically low levels of this finite resource, diabetes is formed.

Lower Cholesterol and Blood Pressure

Cholesterol and triglyceride levels maintain, or ruin, your arterial health. If your arteries are clogged up with cholesterol, they cannot efficiently transfer blood through your system, which in some cases even results in heart attacks. The keto diet keeps all of these levels at an optimal level, so that they do not interfere with your body's normal functioning.

Slow Cookers

Slow cookers are not new appliances in the culinary world. They have been around for decades; you might even have fond memories from your childhood of your parents serving your favorite dinner out of one. Slow cookers are very versatile because the cooking environment works the same no matter the cuisine. Knowing what slow cookers can and can't do is important for planning your meals, especially for a diet like keto.

Some of the reasons to use a slow cooker include:

Enhances flavor: Cooking ingredients over several hours with spices, herbs, and other seasonings creates vegetables and proteins that burst with delicious flavors. This slow process allows the flavors to mellow and deepen for an enhanced eating experience.

Saves time: Cooking at home takes a great deal of time: prepping, sautéing, stirring, turning the heat up and down, and watching the meal so that it does not over- or undercook. If you're unable to invest the time, you might find yourself reaching for convenience foods instead of healthy choices. Slow cookers allow you to do other activities while the meal cooks. You can put your ingredients in the slow cooker in the morning and come home to a perfectly cooked meal.

Convenient: Besides the time-saving aspect, using a slow cooker can free up the stove and oven for other dishes. This can be very convenient for large holiday meals or when you want to serve a side dish and entrée as well as a delectable dessert. Clean up is simple when you use the slow cooker for messy meals because most inserts are nonstick or are easily cleaned with a little soapy water, and each meal is prepared in either just the machine or using one additional vessel to sauté ingredients. There is no wide assortment of pots, pans, and baking dishes to contend with at the end of the day.

Low heat production: If you have ever cooked dinner on a scorching summer afternoon, you will appreciate the low amount of heat produced by a slow cooker. Even after eight hours of operation, slow cookers do not heat up your kitchen and you will not be sweating over the hot stovetop. Slow cookers use about a third of the energy of conventional cooking methods, just a little more energy than a traditional light bulb.

Supports healthy eating: Cooking your food at high heat can reduce the nutrition profile of your foods, breaking down and removing the majority of vitamins, minerals, and antioxidants while producing unhealthy chemical compounds that can contribute to disease. Low-heat cooking retains all the goodness that you want for your diet.

Saves Money: Slow cookers save you money because of the low amount of electricity they use and because the best ingredients for slow cooking are the less expensive cuts of beef and heartier inexpensive vegetables. Tougher cuts of meat—brisket, chuck, shanks—break down beautifully to fork-tender goodness. Another cost-saving benefit is that most 6-quart slow cookers will produce enough of a recipe to stretch your meals over at least two days. Leftovers are one of the best methods for saving money.

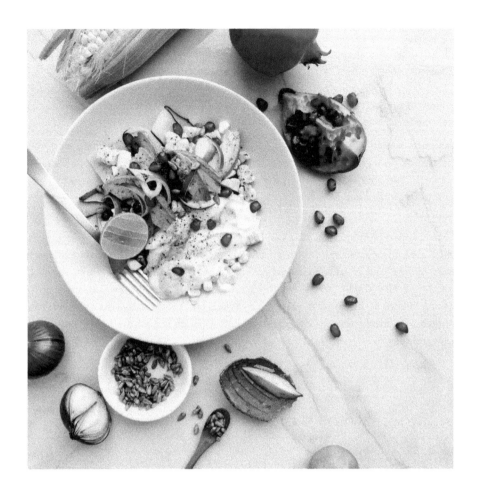

BREAKFAST

1. Eggplant Pate with Breadcrumbs

Preparation Time: 27 minutes

Cooking time: 6 hours

Servings: 15

Ingredients:

- 5 medium eggplants
- 2 sweet green pepper
- 1cup bread crumbs
- 1teaspoon salt
- 1tablespoon sugar
- 1/2cup tomato paste
- 2 yellow onion
- 1tablespoon minced garlic
- 1/4chili pepper
- 1teaspoon olive oil
- 1teaspoon kosher salt
- 1tablespoon mayonnaise

Directions:

1. Peel the eggplants and chop them.
2. Sprinkle the chopped eggplants with the salt and let sit for 10 minutes.

3. Meanwhile, combine the tomato paste with the kosher salt and sugar.

4. Add minced garlic and mayonnaise. Whisk carefully. Then, peel the onions and chop.

5. Spray the slow cooker bowl with the olive oil. Add the chopped onions.

6. Strain the chopped eggplants to get rid of the eggplant juice and transfer the strained eggplants into the slow cooker bowl as well. After this, add the tomato paste mixture.

7. Chop the chili pepper and sweet green peppers and add them to the slow cooker too. Stir the mixture inside the slow cooker carefully and close the lid.

8. Cook the dish for 6 hours on LOW. When the time is done, transfer the prepared mix into a bowl and blend it .

9. Sprinkle the prepared plate with the bread crumbs. Enjoy!

Nutrition: Calories 83 Fat 1 Carbs 1.4 Protein 18

2. <u>Red Beans with the Sweet Peas</u>

Preparation Time: 21 minutes

Cooking time: 6 hours

Servings: 5

Ingredients:

- 1cup red beans, dried
- 3 chicken stock
- 3tablespoon tomato paste
- onion
- 1teaspoon salt
- 1 chili pepper
- 1teaspoon sriracha
- 1tablespoon butter
- 1teaspoon turmeric
- 1cup green peas

Directions:

1. Place the red beans in water for 5 hours in advance.
2. After this, strain the red beans and put them in the slow cooker.
3. Add the chicken stock, salt, and turmeric.
4. Close and cook the red beans for 4 hours on HIGH.
5. Meanwhile, peel the onion and slice it. Combine the sliced onion with the tomato paste, sriracha, and butter. Chop the chili pepper and add it to the onion mixture.

6. When the time is done, open the slow cooker lid and add the onion mixture.

7. Stir it very carefully and close the slow cooker lid. Cook the dish for 1 hour more on Low.

8. Stir the red beans mixture carefully again and add the green peas. Cook the dish on LOW for 1 more hour. After this, stir the dish gently and serve. Enjoy!

Nutrition: Calories 190 Fat 3 Carbs 1.8 Protein 11

3. Nutritious Burrito Bowl

Preparation Time: 18 minutes

Cooking time: 7 hours

Servings: 6

Ingredients:

- 10 oz.. chicken breast
- 1tablespoon chili flakes
- 1teaspoon salt
- 1teaspoon onion powder
- 1teaspoon minced garlic
- 1/2cup white beans, canned
- 1/4cup green peas
- 1cup chicken stock
- 1/2 avocado, pitted
- 1teaspoon ground black pepper

Directions:

1. Put the chicken breast in the slow cooker.
2. Sprinkle the chicken breast with the chili flakes, salt, onion powder, minced garlic, and ground black pepper. Add the chicken stock.
3. Close and cook the dish for 2 hours on HIGH.
4. After this, open the slow cooker lid and add the white beans and green peas.

5. Mix and close the lid. Cook the dish for 5 hours more on LOW.

6. When the time is done, remove the meat, white beans, and green peas from the slow cooker. Transfer the white beans and green peas to the serving bowls.

7. Shred the chicken breast and add it to the serving bowls too.

8. After this, peel the avocado and chop it. Sprinkle the prepared burrito bowls with the chopped avocado. Enjoy!

Nutrition: Calories 192 Fat 7 Carbs 1.3 Protein 11

4. Quinoa Curry

Preparation Time: 20 minutes

Cooking time: 9 hours

Servings: 7

Ingredients:

- 8oz.. potato
- 7oz.. cauliflower
- 1cup onion, chopped
- 7oz.. chickpea, canned
- 1cup tomatoes, chopped
- 13oz.. almond milk
- 3cup chicken stock
- 8tablespoon quinoa
- 1/3tablespoon miso
- 1teaspoon minced garlic
- 2teaspoon curry paste

Directions:

1. Peel the potatoes and chop them.
2. Put the chopped potatoes, onion, and tomatoes into the slow cooker. Combine the miso, chicken stock, and curry paste.
3. Whisk the mixture until the ingredients are dissolved in the chicken stock. Pour the chicken stock in the slow cooker too.
4. Separate the cauliflower into the florets.

5. Add the cauliflower florets and the chickpeas in the slow cooker.

6. Add the almond milk, quinoa, and minced garlic.

7. Close and cook the dish on LOW for 9 hours.

8. When the dish is cooked, chill it and then mix it gently.

9. Transfer the prepared curry quinoa to the bowls. Enjoy!

Nutrition: Calories 262 Fat 4 Carbs 1.8 Protein 12

5. Ham Pitta Pockets

Preparation Time: 14 minutes

Cooking time: 1.5 minutes

Servings: 6

Ingredients

- 6pita breads, sliced
- 7oz.. mozzarella, sliced
- 1teaspoon minced garlic
- 7oz.. ham, sliced
- 1big tomato, sliced
- 1tablespoon mayo
- 1tablespoon heavy cream

Directions:

1. Preheat the slow cooker on HIGH for 30 minutes.
2. Combine the mayo, heavy cream, and minced garlic.
3. After this, fill the pitta bread with the sliced moz.zarella, tomato, and ham.
4. Wrap the pita bread in foil and place them in the slow cooker.
5. Close and cook the dish for 1.5 hours on HIGH.
6. Then discard the foil and serve the prepared pita pockets immediately. Enjoy!

Nutrition: Calories 273 Fat 3 Carbs 1.0 Protein 10

6. Breakfast Meatloaf

Preparation Time: 18 minutes

Cooking time: 7 hours

Servings: 8

Ingredients:

- 12oz.. ground beef
- 1teaspoon salt
- 1teaspoon ground coriander
- 1tablespoon ground mustard
- 1/4teaspoon ground chili pepper
- 6oz.. white bread
- 1/2cup milk
- 1teaspoon ground black pepper
- 3tablespoon tomato sauce

Directions:

1. Chop the white bread and combine it with the milk.
2. Stir then set aside for 3 minutes.
3. Meanwhile, combine the ground beef, salt, ground coriander, ground mustard, ground chili pepper, and ground black pepper.
4. Stir the white bread mixture carefully and add it to the ground beef. Cover the slow cooker bowl with foil.
5. Shape the meatloaf and place the uncooked meatloaf in the slow cooker then spread it with the tomato sauce.
6. Close the slow cooker lid and cook

7. Slice the prepared meatloaf and serve. Enjoy!

Nutrition: Calories 214 Fat 14 Carbs 1.2 Protein 9

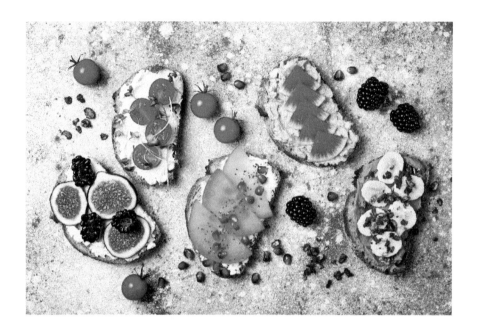

LUNCH

7. Mexican Warm Salad

Preparation time: 26 minutes

Cooking time: 10 hours

Servings: 10

Ingredients:

- 1cup black beans
- 1cup sweet corn, froz.en
- 3 tomatoes
- 1/2 cup fresh dill
- chili pepper
- 7 oz.. chicken fillet
- 5 oz.. Cheddar cheese
- 4tablespoons mayonnaise
- 1teaspoon minced garlic
- 1cup lettuce
- 5cups chicken stock
- 1cucumber

Directions:

1. Put the chicken fillet, sweet corn, black beans, and chicken stock in the slow cooker.

2. Close the slow cooker lid and cook the mixture on LOW for 10 hours.

3. When the time is done remove the mixture from the slow cooker.

4. Shred the chicken fillet with 2 forks. Chill the mixture until room temperature.

5. Chop the lettuce roughly. Chop the cucumber and tomatoes.

6. Place the lettuce, cucumber, and tomatoes on a large serving plate.

7. After this, shred Cheddar cheese and chop the chili pepper.

8. Add the chili pepper to the serving plate too.

9. After this, add the chicken mixture on the top of the salad.

10. Sprinkle the salad with the mayonnaise, minced garlic, and shredded cheese. Enjoy the salad immediately.

Nutrition: Calories 182, Fat 7.8, Fiber 2, Carbs 1.6, Protein 9

8. Hot Chorizo Salad

Preparation time: 20 minutes

Cooking time: 4 hours 30 minutes

Servings: 6

Ingredients:

- 8 oz.. chorizo
- 1teaspoon olive oil
- 1teaspoon cayenne pepper
- 1teaspoon chili flakes
- 1teaspoon ground black pepper
- 1teaspoon onion powder
- 2garlic cloves
- 3tomatoes
- 1cup lettuce
- 1cup fresh dill
- 1teaspoon oregano
- 3tablespoons crushed cashews

Directions:

1. Chop the chorizo sausages roughly and place them in the slow cooker.
2. Cook the sausages for 4 hours on HIGH.
3. Meanwhile, combine the cayenne pepper, chili flakes, ground black pepper, and onion powder together in a shallow bowl.

4. Chop the tomatoes roughly and add them to the slow cooker after 4 hours. Cook the mixture for 30 minutes more on HIGH.

5. Chop the fresh dill and combine it with oregano.

6. When the chorizo sausage mixture is cooked, place it in a serving bowl. Tear the lettuce and add it in the bowl too.

7. After this, peel the garlic cloves and slice them.

8. Add the sliced garlic cloves in the salad bowl too.

9. Then sprinkle the salad with the spice mixture, olive oil, fresh dill mixture, and crush cashew. Mix the salad carefully. Enjoy!

Nutrition: Calories 249, Fat 19.8, Fiber 2, Carbs 1.69, Protein 11

9. Stuffed Eggplants

Preparation time: 20 minutes

Cooking time: 8 hours

Servings: 4

Ingredients:

- 4medium eggplants
- 1cup rice, half cooked
- 1/2cup chicken stock
- 1teaspoon salt
- 1teaspoon paprika
- 1/2cup fresh cilantro
- 3tablespoons tomato sauce
- 1teaspoon olive oil

Directions:

1. Wash the eggplants carefully and remove the flesh from them.
2. Then combine the rice with the salt, paprika, and tomato sauce.
3. Chop the fresh cilantro and add it to the rice mixture.
4. Then fill the prepared eggplants with the rice mixture.
5. Pour the chicken stock and olive oil in the slow cooker.
6. Add the stuffed eggplants and close the slow cooker lid.
7. Cook the dish on LOW for 8 hours. When the eggplants are done, chill them little and serve immediately. Enjoy!

Nutrition: Calories 277, Fat 9.1, Fiber 24, Carbs 1.92, Protein 11

10.Light Lunch Quiche

Preparation time: 21 minutes

Cooking time: 4 hours 25 minutes

Servings: 7

Ingredients:

- 7oz.. pie crust
- 1/4cup broccoli
- 1/3cup sweet peas
- 1/4cup heavy cream
- 2tablespoons flour
- 3eggs
- 4oz.. Romano cheese, shredded
- 1teaspoon cilantro
- 1teaspoon salt
- 1/4cup spinach
- 1tomato

Directions:

1. Cover the inside of the slow cooker bowl with parchment.
2. Put the pie crust inside and flatten it well with your fingertips.
3. Chop the broccoli and combine it with sweet peas. Combine the heavy cream, flour, cilantro, and salt together. Stir the liquid until smooth.

4. Then beat the eggs into the heavy cream liquid and mix it with a hand mixer. When you get a smooth mix, combine it with the broccoli.

5. Chop the spinach and add it to the mix. Chop the tomato and add it to the mix too. Pour the prepared mixture into the pie crust slowly.

6. Close the slow cooker lid and cook the quiche for 4 hours on HIGH.

7. After 4 hours, sprinkle the quiche surface with the shredded cheese and cook the dish for 25 minutes more. Serve the prepared quiche! Enjoy!

Nutrition: Calories 287, Fat 18.8, Fiber 1, Carbs 1.1, Protein 11

11. Chicken Open Sandwich

Preparation time: 15 minutes

Cooking time: 8 hours

Servings: 4

Ingredients:

- 7oz.. chicken fillet
- 1teaspoon cayenne pepper
- 5oz.. mashed potato, cooked
- 6tablespoons chicken gravy
- 4slices French bread, toasted
- 2teaspoons mayo
- 1cup water

Directions:

1. Put the chicken fillet in the slow cooker and sprinkle it with the cayenne pepper.
2. Add water and chicken gravy. Close the slow cooker lid and cook the chicken for 8 hours on LOW. Then combine the mashed potato with the mayo sauce.
3. Spread toasted French bread with the mashed potato mixture.
4. When the chicken is cooked, cut it into the strips and combine with the remaining gravy from the slow cooker.
5. Place the chicken strips over the mashed potato. Enjoy the open sandwich warm!

Nutrition: Calories 314, Fat 9.7, Fiber 3, Carbs 4.1, Protein 12

12.Onion Lunch Muffins

Preparation time: 15 minutes

Cooking time: 8 hours

Servings: 7

Ingredients:

- 1egg
- 5tablespoons butter, melted
- 1cup flour
- 1/2cup milk
- 1teaspoon baking soda
- 1cup onion, chopped
- 1teaspoon cilantro
- 1/2teaspoon sage
- 1teaspoon apple cider vinegar
- 2cup water
- 1tablespoon chives
- 1teaspoon olive oil

Directions:

1. Beat the egg in the bowl and add melted butter.
2. Add the flour, baking soda, chopped onion, milk, sage, apple cider vinegar, cilantro, and chives. Knead into a dough.
3. After this, spray a muffin form with the olive oil inside. Fill the 1/2 part of every muffin form and place them in the glass jars.
4. After this, pour water in the slow cooker vessel.

5. Place the glass jars with muffins in the slow cooker and close the lid.

6. Cook the muffins for 8 hours on LOW.

7. Check if the muffins are cooked with the help of the toothpick and remove them from the slow cooker. Enjoy the dish warm!

Nutrition: Calories 180, Fat 11, Fiber 1, Carbs 1.28, Protein 4

13. Tuna in Potatoes

Preparation time: 16 minutes

Cooking time: 4 hours

Servings: 8

Ingredients:

- 4large potatoes
- 8oz.. tuna, canned
- 1/2cup cream cheese
- 4oz.. Cheddar cheese
- 1garlic clove
- 1teaspoon onion powder
- 1/2teaspoon salt
- 1teaspoon ground black pepper
- 1teaspoon dried dill

Directions:

1. Wash the potatoes carefully and cut them into the halves.
2. Wrap the potatoes in the foil and place in the slow cooker. Close the slow cooker lid and cook the potatoes on HIGH for 2 hours.
3. Meanwhile, peel the garlic clove and mince it. Combine the minced garlic clove with the cream cheese, tuna, salt, ground black pepper, onion powder, and dill.
4. Then shred Cheddar cheese and add it to the mixture.
5. Mix it carefully until homogenous.

6. When the time is over – remove the potatoes from the slow cooker and discard the foil only from the flat surface of the potatoes.

7. Then take the fork and mash the flesh of the potato halves gently. Add the tuna mixture in the potato halves and return them back in the slow cooker.

8. Cook the potatoes for 2 hours more on HIGH. Enjoy!

Nutrition: Calories 247, Fat 5.9, Fiber 4, Carbs 3.31, Protein 14

14. Banana Lunch Sandwiches

Preparation time: 15 minutes

Cooking time: 2 hours

Servings: 4

Ingredients:

- 2 banana
- 8 oz.. French toast slices, froz.en
- 1tablespoon peanut butter
- 1/4teaspoon ground cinnamon
- 5oz.. Cheddar cheese, sliced
- 1/4teaspoon turmeric

Directions:

1. Peel the bananas and slice them.
2. Spread the French toast slices with the peanut butter well. Combine the ground cinnamon with the turmeric and stir the mixture. Sprinkle the French toasts with the spice mixture.
3. Then make the layer of the sliced bananas on the toasts and add the sliced cheese.
4. Cover the toast with the second part of the toast to make the sandwich.
5. Place the banana sandwiches in the slow cooker and cook them on HIGH for 2 hours.
6. Serve the prepared banana sandwiches hot. Enjoy!

Nutrition: Calories 248, Fat 7.5, Fiber 2, Carbs 3.74 Protein 10

15. Parmesan Potato with Dill

Preparation time: 17 minutes

Cooking time: 4 hours

Servings: 5

Ingredients:

- 1-pound small potato
- 1/2 cup fresh dill
- 7 oz.. Parmesan
- 1 teaspoon rosemary
- 1 teaspoon thyme
- 1 cup water
- 1/4 teaspoon chili flakes
- 3 tablespoon cream
- 1 teaspoon salt

Directions:

1. Peel the potatoes and put them in the slow cooker.
2. Add water, salt, thyme, rosemary, and chili flakes.
3. Close the slow cooker lid and cook the potato for 2 hours on HIGH.
4. Meanwhile, shred Parmesan cheese and chop the fresh dill. When the time is done, sprinkle the potato with the cream and fresh dill. Stir it carefully.
5. Add shredded Parmesan cheese and close the slow cooker lid. Cook the potato on HIGH for 2 hours more.

6. Then open the slow cooker lid and do not stir the potato anymore. Gently transfer the dish to the serving plates. Enjoy!

Nutrition: Calories 235, Fat 3.9, Fiber 2, Carbs 2.26, Protein 1

16. Light Taco Soup

Preparation time: 24 minutes

Cooking time: 7 hours

Servings: 5

Ingredients:

- 7oz.. ground chicken
- 1/2teaspoon sesame oil
- 3cup vegetable stock
- 3oz.. yellow onion
- 1cup tomato, canned
- 3tomatoes
- 5 oz.. corn kernels
- 1jalapeno pepper, sliced
- 1/2cup white beans, drained
- 3tablespoon taco seasoning
- 1/4teaspoon salt
- 3 oz.. black olives, sliced
- 5 corn tortillas, for serving

Directions:

1. Peel the onion and dice it. Chop the fresh and canned tomatoes.

2. Place the ground chicken, sesame oil, vegetable stock, diced onion, chopped tomatoes, sliced black olives, sliced jalapeno pepper, and corn in the slow cooker.

3. Add the white beans, taco seasoning, and salt.

4. Stir the soup mixture gently and close the slow cooker lid.

5. Cook the soup for 7 hours on LOW. Meanwhile, cut the corn tortillas into the strips and bake them in the preheated to 365 F oven for 10 minutes.

6. When the soup is cooked, ladle it into the serving bowls and sprinkle with the baked corn tortilla strips. Enjoy!

Nutrition: Calories 328, Fat 9.6, Fiber 10, Carbs 4.19, Protein 18

17.Slow Cooker Risotto

Preparation time: 20 minutes

Cooking time: 3 hours 30 minutes

Servings: 6

Ingredients:

- 7 oz.. Parmigiano-Reggiano
- 2cup chicken broth
- 1teaspoon olive oil
- 1onion, chopped
- 1/2cup green peas
- 1garlic clove, peeled and sliced
- 2cups long grain rice
- 1/4cup dry wine
- 1teaspoon salt
- 1teaspoon ground black pepper
- 1carrot, chopped
- 1cup beef broth

Directions:

1. Spray a skillet with olive oil.
2. Add the chopped onion and carrot and roast the vegetables for 3 minutes on the medium heat. Then put the seared vegetables in the slow cooker. Toss the long grain rice in the remaining oil and sauté for 1 minute on the high heat.

3. Add the roasted long grain rice and sliced garlic in the slow cooker.

4. Add green peas, dry wine, salt, ground black pepper, and beef broth. After this, add the chicken broth and stir the mixture gently. Close the slow cooker lid and cook the risotto for 3 hours.

5. Then stir the risotto gently.

6. Shred Parmigiano-Reggiano and sprinkle over the risotto. Close the slow cooker lid and cook the dish for 30 minutes more. Enjoy the prepared risotto immediately!

Nutrition: Calories 268, Fat 3, Fiber 4, Carbs 3.34, Protein 7

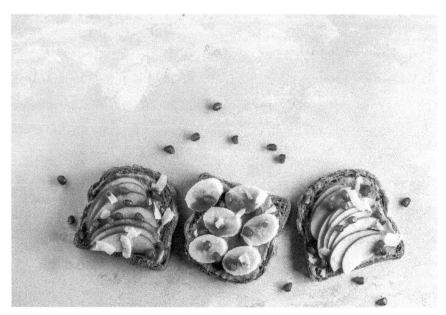

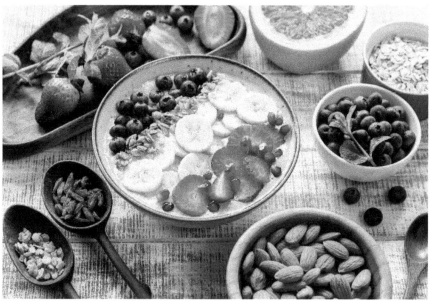

DINNER

18.Chicken Chile Verde

Preparation Time: 12 minutes

Cooking Time: 6 hours

Servings: 9

Ingredients:

- 1/4 teaspoon sea salt

- 2 pounds chopped boneless chicken.

- 3 tablespoons divided butter

- 3 tablespoons neatly chopped & divided cilantro

- 5 minced & divided garlic cloves

- 1 extra tablespoon cilantro, to garnish

- 1 1/2 cups salsa Verde

Directions:

1. Dissolve 2 tablespoons of butter in the slow cooker on high.

2. Add in 4 of the garlic along with 2 tablespoons cilantro, then stir.

3. Use a stovetop, melt 1 tablespoon butter in a big frypan over medium-high heat, and add 1 tablespoon minced garlic and cilantro.

4. Put in the chopped chicken, then sear until all the sides are browned but not cooked through.

5. Add the cilantro, garlic, and butter mixture with browned chicken into the slow cooker.

6. Pour in the salsa Verde and stir together.

7. Cover the slow cooker and cook on high settings for 2 hours, then reduce to a low setting for 3-4 extra hours.

8. Serve the chicken Verde in a lettuce cup or over cauliflower rice.

Nutrition: Calories: 140 Carbs: 5 g Fat: 4g Protein: 18g

19. Cauliflower & Ham Potato Stew

Preparation Time: 5 minutes

Cooking Time: 4 hours

Servings: 6

Ingredients:

- 1/4 teaspoon salt
- 1/4 cup heavy cream
- 1/2 teaspoon onion powder
- 1/2 teaspoon garlic powder
- 3 cups diced ham
- 4 garlic cloves
- 8 oz. grated cheddar cheese
- 14 1/2 oz. chicken broth
- 16 oz. bag frozen cauliflower florets
- A dash of pepper

Directions:

1. Put all the items except the cauliflower inside the slow cooker and mix.
2. Cover the slow cooker, then cook for 4 hours on a high setting.
3. Once done, add in the cauliflower and cook for an extra 30 minutes on high. Serve and enjoy.

Nutrition: Calories: 71 Carbs: 2g Fat: 4g Protein: 6g

20.   **Beef Dijon**

Preparation Time: 15 minutes

Cooking Time: 5 hours

Servings: 4

Ingredients:

- 6 oz. Small round steaks
- 2 tbsp. of each:
- Steak seasoning - to taste
- Avocado oil
- Peanut oil
- Balsamic vinegar/dry sherry
- Large chopped green onions/small chopped onions for the garnish - extra
- 1/4 c. whipping cream
- 1cup. fresh crimini mushrooms - sliced
- 1tbsp. Dijon mustard

Directions:

1. Warm up the oils using the high heat setting on the stove top. Flavor each of the steaks with pepper and arrange to a skillet.
2. Cook two to three minutes per side until done.
3. Place into the slow cooker. Pour in the skillet drippings, half of the mushrooms, and the onions.
4. Cook on the low setting for four hours.

5. When the cooking time is done, scoop out the onions, mushrooms, and steaks to a serving platter.

6. In a separate dish - whisk together the mustard, balsamic vinegar, whipping cream, and the steak drippings from the slow cooker.

7. Empty the gravy into a gravy server and pour over the steaks.

8. Enjoy with some brown rice, riced cauliflower, or potatoes.

Nutrition: Calories: 535 Carbs: 5.0 g Fat: 40 g Protein: 39 g

21.Cabbage & Corned Beef

Preparation Time: 10 minutes

Cooking Time: 8 hours

Servings: 10

Ingredients:

- 1 lb. corned beef
- 1 large head of cabbage
- 1cup water
- 1 celery bunch
- 1 small onion
- 2 carrots
- 1/2tsp.Ground mustard
- 1/2tsp.Ground coriander
- 1/2tsp.Ground marjoram
- 1/2tsp.Black pepper
- 1/2tsp.Salt
- 1/2tsp.Ground thyme
- Allspice

Directions:

1. Dice the carrots, onions, and celery and toss them into the cooker. Pour in the water.
2. Combine the spices, rub the beef, and arrange in the cooker. Secure the lid and cook on low for seven hours.

3. Remove the top layer of cabbage. Wash and cut it into quarters until ready to cook. When the beef is done, add the cabbage, and cook for one hour on the low setting.

4. Serve and enjoy.

Nutrition: Calories: 583 Carbs: 1.3 g Fat: 40 g Protein: 42 g

22. **Chipotle Baracoa**

Preparation Time: 20 minutes

Cooking Time: 4 hours

Servings: 9

Ingredients:

- 1/2 cup beef/chicken broth
- 4tsp chilies
- 1lb. chuck roast/beef brisket
- Minced garlic cloves
- 2tbsp.Lime juice
- 2tbsp.Apple cider vinegar
- 1tsps. of each:
- 1tsps. Sea salt
- 2 tsps. Cumin
- 1 tbsp. dried oregano
- 1 tsp. black pepper
- whole bay leaves
- Optional: 1/2 t. ground cloves

Directions:

1. Mix the chilies in the sauce, and add the broth, garlic, ground cloves, pepper, cumin, salt, vinegar, and lime juice in a blender, mixing until smooth.

2. Chop the beef into two-inch chunks and toss it in the slow cooker. Empty the puree on top. Toss in the two bay leaves.

3. Cook four to six hrs. On the high setting or eight to ten using the low setting.

4. Dispose of the bay leaves when the meat is done.

5. Shred and stir into the juices to simmer for five to ten minutes.

Nutrition: Calories: 242 Net Carbs: 2 g Fat: 11 g Protein: 32 g

23.   <u>Corned Beef Cabbage Rolls</u>

Preparation Time: 25 minutes

Cooking Time: 6 hours

Servings: 5

Ingredients:

- 1/2 lb.. corned beef
- large savoy cabbage leaves
- 1/4cupWhite wine
- 1/4cupCoffee
- large lemon
- 1 med. sliced onion
- 1tbsp.Rendered bacon fat
- 1tbsp.Erythritol
- 1tbsp.Yellow mustard
- 2tbsp.Kosher salt
- 2tbsp.Worcestershire sauce
- 1/4tsp.Cloves
- 1/4tsp Allspice
- 1/4tsp large bay leaf
- 1tsp.Mustard seeds
- 1tsp.Whole peppercorns
- 1tsp.1/2 t. red pepper flakes

Directions:

1. Add the liquids, spices, and corned beef into the cooker. Cook six hours on the low setting.

2. Prepare a pot of boiling water.

3. When the time is up, add the leaves along with the sliced onion to the water for two to three minutes.

4. Transfer the leaves to a cold-water bath - blanching them for three to four minutes. Continue boiling the onion.

5. Use a paper towel to dry the leaves. Add the onions and beef. Roll up the cabbage leaves.

6. Drizzle with freshly squeezed lemon juice.

Nutrition: Calories: 481.4 Carbs: 4.2 g Protein: 34.87 g Fat: 25.38 g

24. Cube Steak

Preparation Time: 15 minutes

Cooking Time: 8 hours

Servings: 8

Ingredients:

- 28 oz.. Cubed steaks
- 1 3/4 t. adobo seasoning/garlic salt
- 1 can (8 oz..) tomato sauce
- 1 c. water
- Black pepper to taste
- 1/2 med. onion
- 1 small red pepper
- 1/3 c. green pitted olives
- 2 tbsp.. brine

Directions:

1. Slice the peppers and onions into 1/4-inch strips.
2. Sprinkle the steaks with the pepper and garlic salt as needed and place them in the cooker.
3. Fold in the peppers and onion along with the water, sauce, and olives (with the liquid/brine from the jar).
4. Close the lid. Prepare using the low-temperature setting for eight hours.

Nutrition: Calories: 154 Carbs: 4 g Protein: 23.5 g Fat: 5.5 g

25. <u>Ragu</u>

Preparation Time: 10 minutes

Cooking Time: 8 hours

Servings: 2

Ingredients:

- 1/4Carrot
- 1/4Rib of celery
- 1/4Onion
- 1/41 minced garlic clove
- 1/2 lb.. top-round lean beef
- 3oz.Diced tomatoes
- 3oz.Crushed tomatoes
- 2tsp.. beef broth
- 11/4tsp.Chopped fresh thyme
- 11/4tsp.Minced fresh rosemary
- 1bay leaf
- Pepper & Salt to taste

Directions:

1. Place the prepared celery, garlic, onion, and carrots into the slow cooker.
2. Trim away the fat, and add the meat to the slow cooker. Sprinkle with the salt and pepper
3. Stir in the rest of the ingredients.

4. Prepare on the low setting for six to eight hours. Enjoy any way you choose.

Nutrition: Calories: 224 Carbs: 5 g Protein: 27 g Fat: 9 g

26.   Ropa Vieja

Preparation Time: 15 minutes

Cooking Time: 8 hours

Servings: 6

Ingredients:

- 2 lb.. flank steak – remove fat
- 1tsp.Yellow pepper
- 1Thinly sliced onion
- 1Green pepper
- 1Bay leaf
- 1/4tsp. salt
- 3/4Oregano
- 3/4-fat beef broth
- 3/41 tbsp.. tomato paste
- Cooking spray

Directions:

1. Prepare the slow cooker with the spray or use a liner and combine all of the fixings.
2. Stir everything together and prepare using low for eight hours.
3. Top it off with your chosen garnishes.

Nutrition: Calories: 257 Carbs: 4 g Fat: 10 g Protein: 35 g

27. Spinach Soup

Preparation Time: 15 minutes

Cooking Time: 6-8 hours

Servings: 4

Ingredients:

- 2 pounds spinach
- 1/4 cup cream cheese
- 1 onion, diced
- 2 cups heavy cream
- 1 garlic clove, minced
- 2 cups water
- salt, pepper, to taste

Directions:

1. Pour water into the slow cooker. Add spinach, salt, and pepper.
2. Add cream cheese, onion, garlic, and heavy cream.
3. Close the lid and cook on Low for 6-8 hours.
4. Puree soup with blender and serve.

Nutrition: Calories: 322 Fats: 28.2g Carbs: 1.1g Protein: 12.2g

28. Mashed Cauliflower with Herbs

Preparation Time: 15 minutes

Cooking Time: 3-6 hours

Servings: 4

Ingredients:

- 1 cauliflower head, cut into florets
- 3 garlic cloves, peeled
- 1/2 teaspoon fresh rosemary, chopped
- 1/2 teaspoon fresh thyme, chopped
- 1/2 teaspoon fresh sage, chopped
- 1/2 teaspoon fresh parsley, chopped
- 1 cup vegetable broth
- 2 cups water
- 2 tablespoons, ghee
- Salt, pepper, to taste

Directions:

1. Pour broth into the slow cooker, add cauliflower florets.
2. Add water, it should cover the cauliflower.
3. Close the lid and cook on Low for 6 hours or on High for 3 hours.
4. Once cooked, drain water from the slow cooker.
5. Add herbs, salt, pepper, and ghee, puree with a blender.

Nutrition: Calories 115 Fats 12g carbs 4.7g Protein 6.2g

29. Kale Quiche

Preparation Time: 15 minutes Cooking Time: 3-5 hours

Servings: 3

Ingredients:

- 1 cup almond milk
- 2 eggs
- 1 cup Carb Quick Baking Mix
- 2 cups spinach, chopped
- 1/2 bell pepper, chopped
- 2 cups fresh baby kale, chopped
- 1 teaspoon garlic, chopped
- 1/3 cup fresh basil, chopped
- Salt, pepper, to taste
- 1 tablespoon olive oil

Directions:

1. Add oil to a slow cooker or use a cooking spray.
2. Beat eggs into a slow cooker; add almond milk and Baking Mix, mix to combine.
3. Add spinach, bell pepper, garlic, and basil, stir to combine.
4. Close the lid and cook on Low for 5 hours or on High for 3 hours.
5. Make sure the quiche is done, check the center with a toothpick, it should be dry.

Nutrition: Calories: 273 Fats: 24.4g Carbs: 5.g Protein: 10.5g

MEAT RECIPES

30. Peachy Sweet Pork

Preparation time: 10 minutes

Cooking time: 7 hours

Servings: 6

Ingredients:

- sweet potatoes
- peach, pitted, peeled, and diced
- ½ cup water
- ½ cup peach preserves jelly
- 1 teaspoon cumin
- 2 pork loins, about 1½ pounds each
- Salt and Pepper
- Cooking spray

Directions:

1 Spray slow cooker with nonstick spray.

2 Place pork in a slow cooker. Season with salt and pepper.

3 Place the sweet potatoes around the pork.

4 Stir together the peach preserves, water, and cumin. Pour the sauce over the pork and potatoes.

5 Cook on LOW for 7 hours.

Nutrition: calories 516, fat 29, carbs 18, protein 44

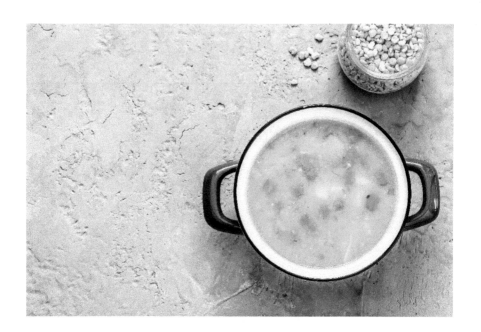

POULTRY

31. Rotisserie Chicken

Preparation Time: 10 minutes

Cooking Time: 8 hours 5 minutes

Servings: 10

Ingredients:

- 1 organic whole chicken
- 1 tablespoon of olive oil
- 1 teaspoon of thyme
- 1 teaspoon of rosemary
- 1 teaspoon of garlic, granulated
- salt and pepper

Directions:

1. Start by seasoning the chicken with all the herbs and spices.
2. Broil this seasoned chicken for 5 minutes in the oven until golden brown.
3. Place this chicken in the Slow cooker.
4. Cover it and cook for 8 hours on Low Settings.
5. Serve warm.

Nutrition: Calories 301 Total Fat 12.2 g Saturated Fat 2.4 g Cholesterol 110 mg Total Carbs 2.5 g Fiber 0.9 g Sugar 1.4 g Sodium 276 mg Potassium 231 mg Protein 28.8 g

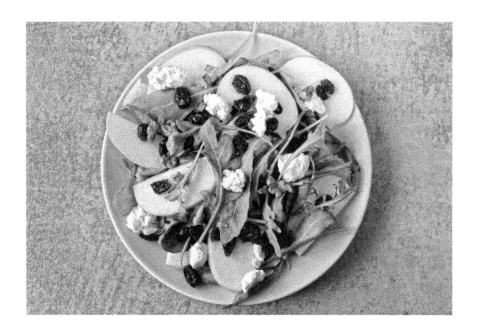

SIDE DISH RECIPES

32. Garlic Carrots Mix

Preparation time: 15 minutes

Cooking time: 4 Hours

Servings: 2

Ingredients

- 1 pound carrots, sliced
- 2 garlic cloves, minced
- 1 red onion, chopped
- 1 tablespoon olive oil
- ½ cup tomato sauce
- A pinch of salt and black pepper
- ½ teaspoon oregano, dried
- 2 teaspoons lemon zest, grated
- 1 tablespoon lemon juice
- 1 tablespoon chives, chopped

Directions:

1. In your Slow cooker, mix the carrots with the garlic, onion and then add the other Ingredients, toss, put the lid on and cook on Low for 4 hours.
2. Divide the mix between plates and serve.

Nutrition: calories 219, fat 8, fiber 4, carbs 8, protein 17

33.   Marjoram Rice Mix

Preparation time: 15 minutes

Cooking time: 6 Hours

Servings: 2

Ingredients

- 1 cup wild rice
- 2 cups chicken stock
- 1 carrot, peeled and grated
- 2 tablespoons marjoram, chopped
- 1 tablespoon olive oil
- A pinch of salt and black pepper
- 1 tablespoon green onions, chopped

Directions:

1. In your Slow cooker, mix the rice with the stock and after that add the other Ingredients, toss, put the lid on and cook on Low for 6 hours.
2. Divide between plates and serve.

Nutrition: calories 200, fat 2, fiber 3, carbs 7, protein 5

VEGETABLES

34. Vegan Cream of Mushroom Soup

Preparation time: 15 minutes

Cooking time: 1 hour & 40 minutes

Servings: 2

Ingredients

- `¼ tsp sea salt
- `½ diced yellow onion
- `½ tsp. extra-virgin olive oil
- `1 ½ C. chopped white mushrooms
- `1 2/3 C. unsweetened almond milk
- `1 tsp. onion powder
- `2 C. cauliflower florets

Directions:

1. Add cauliflower, pepper, salt, onion powder, and milk to slow cooker. Stir and set to cook on high 1 hour.

2. With olive oil, sauté onions and mushrooms together 8 to 10 minutes till softened.

3. Allow cauliflower mixture to cool off a bit and add to blender. Blend until smooth. Then blend in mushroom mixture.

4. Pour back into the slow cooker and heat 30 minutes.

Nutrition: Calories: 281 Carbs: 3g Fat: 16g Protein: 11g

35.   <u>Creamy Curry Sauce Noodle Bowl</u>

Preparation time: 15 minutes

Cooking time: 2 hours

Servings: 4

Ingredients

- `½ head chopped cauliflower
- `1 diced red bell pepper
- `1 pack of Kanten Noodles
- `2 chopped carrots
- `2 handfuls of mixed greens
- `Chopped cilantro
- `Curry Sauce:
- `¼ C. avocado oil mayo
- `¼ C. water
- `¼ tsp./ ginger
- `½ tsp. pepper
- `1 ½ tsp. coriander
- `1 tsp. cumin
- `1 tsp turmeric
- `2 tbsp. apple cider vinegar
- `2 tbsp. avocado oil
- `2 tsp. curry powder

Directions:

1. Add all Ingredients, minus curry sauce components, to your slow cooker. Set to cook on high 1-2 hours.

2. In the meantime, add all of the curry sauce Ingredients to a blender. Puree until smooth.

3. Pour over veggie and noodle mixture. Stir well to coat.

Nutrition: Calories: 110 Carbs: 1g Fat: 9g Protein: 7g

36. Spinach Artichoke Casserole

Preparation time: 15 minutes Cooking time: 4 hours

Servings: 10

Ingredients

- `½ tsp. pepper
- `¾ C. coconut flour
- `¾ C. unsweetened almond milk
- `1 C. grated parmesan cheese
- `1 tbsp. baking powder
- `1 tsp. salt
- `3 minced garlic cloves
- `5-ounces chopped spinach
- `6-ounces chopped artichoke hearts
- `8 eggs

Directions:

1. Grease the inside of your slow cooker.
2. Whisk ½ of parmesan cheese, pepper, salt, garlic, artichoke hearts, spinach, eggs, and almond milk.
3. Add baking powder and coconut flour, combining well.
4. Spread into the slow cooker. Sprinkle with remaining parmesan cheese.
5. Cook within 2 to 3 hours on high, or you can cook 4 to 6 hours on a lower heat setting.

Nutrition: Calories: 141 Carbs: 7g Fat: 9g Protein: 10g

37. Asparagus with Lemon

Preparation time: 15 minutes

Cooking time: 2 hours

Servings: 2

Ingredients

- `1 lb. asparagus spears

- `1 tbsp. lemon juice

Directions:

1. Prepare the seasonings: 2 crushed cloves of garlic and salt and pepper to taste.

2. Put the asparagus spears on the bottom of the slow cooker. Add the lemon juice and the seasonings.

3. Cook on low for 2 hours.

Nutrition: Calories: 78 Fat: 2 g Carbs: 3.7 g Protein: 9 g

38.   Veggie-Noodle Soup

Preparation time: 15 minutes

Cooking time: 8 hours

Servings: 2

Ingredients

- `1/2 cup chopped carrots, chopped
- `1/2 cup chopped celery, chopped
- `1 tsp Italian seasoning
- `7 oz. zucchini, cut spiral
- `2 cups spinach leaves, chopped

Directions:

1. Except for the zucchini and spinach, add all the Ingredients: to the slow cooker.
2. Add 3 cups of water.
3. Cover and cook within 8 hours on low. Add the zucchini and spinach at the last 10 minutes of cooking.

Nutrition: Calories: 56 Fat: 0.5 g Carbs: 0.5 g Protein: 3 g

FISH & SEAFOOD

39. Salmon Soup

Preparation Time: 8 minutes

Cooking time: 3 hours

Servings: 4

Ingredients:

- `2 cups of water
- `1 cup coconut cream
- `1 teaspoon garlic powder
- `2 garlic cloves, chopped
- `1 teaspoon lemongrass
- `½ teaspoon chili flakes
- `8 oz salmon, skinless, boneless, and cubed
- `1 teaspoon salt

Directions:

1 In the slow cooker, mix the water with cream and the other ingredients except the fish and close the lid.

2 Cook the stock for 2 hours on High.

3 After this, open the slow cooker lid and add the salmon.

4 Close the lid and cook the soup for 1 hour on Low.

Nutrition: calories 209, fat 12, carbs 5, protein 7

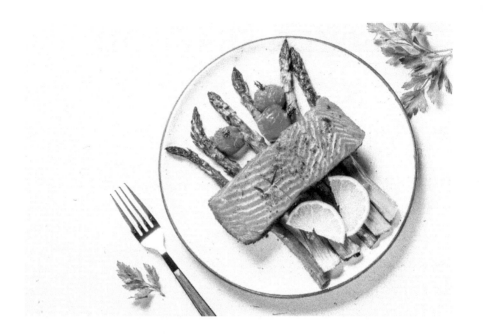

APPETIZERS & SNACKS

40. Radish Spinach Medley

Preparation Time: 10 minutes

Cooking Time: 2 hour

Servings: 2

Ingredients:

- `1lb.. spinach, torn
- `2cups of radishes, sliced
- `A pinch of salt and black pepper
- `1/4cup of vegetable broth
- `1teaspoon of chili powder
- `1tablespoon of parsley, chopped

Directions:

1. Start by throwing all the Ingredients: into the Slow cooker.
2. Cover its lid and cook for 2 hours on Low setting.
3. Once done, remove its lid of the slow cooker carefully.
4. Mix well and garnish as desired.
5. Serve warm.

Nutrition: Calories 244 Fat 24.8 g Sodium 204 mg Carbs 2.1 g Sugar 0.4 g Fiber 0.1 g Protein 24 g

41.Citrus rich Cabbage

Preparation Time: 10 minutes

Cooking Time: 3 hours

Servings: 2

Ingredients:

- `1lb.. green cabbage, shredded
- `1/2cup of chicken stock
- `A pinch of salt and black pepper
- `1tablespoon of lemon juice
- `1tablespoon of chives, diced
- `1tablespoon of lemon zest (grated)

Directions:

1. Start by throwing all the Ingredients: into the Slow cooker.
2. Cover its lid and cook for 3 hours on Low setting.
3. Once done, remove its lid of the slow cooker carefully.
4. Mix well and garnish as desired.
5. Serve warm.

Nutrition: Calories 145 Fat 13.1 g Sodium 35 mg Carbs 4 g Sugar 1.2 g Fiber 1.5 g Protein 3.5 g

42.   Herb Mixed Radish

Preparation Time: 10 minutes

Cooking Time: 3 hours

Servings: 4

Ingredients:

- `3cups of red radishes, halved

- `1/2cup of vegetable broth

- `2tablespoons of basil, diced

- `1tablespoon of oregano, diced

- `1tablespoon of chives, diced

- `1tablespoon of green onion, diced

- `A pinch of salt and black pepper

Directions:

1. Start by throwing all the Ingredients: into the Slow cooker.

2. Cover its lid and cook for 3 hours on Low setting.

3. Once done, remove its lid of the slow cooker carefully.

4. Mix well and garnish as desired.

5. Serve warm.

Nutrition: Calories 266 Fat 26.9 g Sodium 218 mg Carbs 2.5 g Sugar 0.4 g Fiber 0.2 g Protein 4.5 g

43. Creamy Mustard Asparagus

Preparation Time: 10 minutes

Cooking Time: 3 hours

Servings: 2

Ingredients:

- `1lb.. asparagus, trimmed and halved
- `2teaspoons of mustard
- `1/4cup of coconut cream
- `2garlic cloves, minced
- `1tablespoon of chives, diced
- `Salt and black pepper- to taste

Directions:

1. Start by throwing all the Ingredients: into the Slow cooker.
2. Cover its lid and cook for 3 hours on Low setting.
3. Once done, remove its lid of the slow cooker carefully.
4. Mix well and garnish as desired.
5. Serve warm.

Nutrition: Calories 149 Fat 14.5 g Sodium 56 mg Carbs 1.6 g Sugar 0.3 g Fiber 0.2 g Protein 2.6 g

44.   Perfect Eggplant Tapenade

Preparation time: 15 minutes

Cooking time: 9 hours

Servings: 2

Ingredients

- 1cups eggplants, chopped
- 1cup tomatoes, chopped
- garlic cloves, minced
- 2teaspoons capers
- 2teaspoons fresh lemon juice
- 1teaspoon dried basil
- Salt, to taste
- Pinch of ground black pepper

Directions:

1. In a slow cooker, add eggplant, tomatoes, garlic, and capers and mix well.
2. Cook on low, covered, for about 7-9 hours.
3. Uncover the slow cooker and stir in the remaining Ingredients
4. Serve hot.

Nutrition: Calories: 46 Carbohydrates: 10.1g Protein: 2g Fat: 0.4g Sugar: 5g Sodium: 170mg Fiber: 4.2g

45. Swiss Style Cheese Fondue

Preparation time: 15 minutes Cooking time: 3 hours & 10 minutes
Servings: 6

Ingredients

- 1clove garlic, cut in half
- 2½ cups homemade chicken broth
- 1tablespoons fresh lemon juice
- 16ounces Swiss cheese, shredded
- 1ounces Cheddar cheese, shredded
- 1tablespoons almond flour
- Pinch of ground nutmeg
- Pinch of paprika
- Pinch of ground black pepper

Directions:

1. Rub a pan evenly with cut garlic halves. Add broth and place pan over medium heat. Cook until mixture is just beginning to bubble. Adjust to low, then stir in lemon juice.
2. Meanwhile, in a bowl, mix cheeses and flour. Slowly, add cheese mixture to broth, stirring continuously.
3. Cook until cheese mixture becomes thick, stirring continuously. Transfer the cheese mixture to a greased slow cooker and sprinkle with nutmeg, paprika, and black pepper.
4. Cook in the slow cooker on low, covered, for about 1-3 hours.

Nutrition: Calories: 479 Carbohydrates: 6.1g Protein: 32.6g Fat: 36g Sugar: 1.8g Sodium: 700mg Fiber: 0.5g

DESSERT

46. Sweet Potato Brownies

Preparation Time: 50 minutes

Cooking Time 1 h 40 minutes

Serving: 6

Ingredients:

- `600 g sweet potatoes
- `15 dates
- `4 tbsp.. coconut oil (melted)
- `5 tbsp.. honey
- `100 g whole meal spelled flour
- `100 g ground almond
- `1/2 tsp.. salt
- `8 tbsp.. cocoa powder
- `2 tbsp.. almond butter

Directions:

1. Wash, peel, and cut the sweet potatoes into large pieces. Put this in a saucepan with some water and cook for about 20 minutes until the sweet potato is soft.
2. Put the soft sweet potato pieces together with the pitted dates in a food processor and puree to a paste.

3. Mix 2 tablespoons of coconut oil, 4 tablespoons of honey, wholegrain spelled flour, ground almonds, salt and 6 tablespoons of cocoa powder in a large bowl, and knead thoroughly with the sweet potato and date mix. Pour the finished dough into a 26 x 20-centimetre mould lined with baking paper and bake in a preheated oven at 180 ° C (convection: 160 ° C; gas: level 2–3) for about 50 minutes.

4. If no batter sticks to the wooden stick when you pierce the sweet potato brownie, it is ready and can be taken out of the oven. Now the whole thing has to cool for about 15 minutes so that the brownie doesn't fall apart when you lift it out.

5. For the glaze, melt 1 tbsp.. honey, 2 tbsp.. coconut oil, 2 tbsp.. almond butter, and 2 tbsp.. cocoa powder in a small saucepan and stir together. Then cool down to room temperature, for example, in the refrigerator.

6. Before the sweet potato brownie can be glazed, it must be completely cooled—otherwise, the glaze will melt! Then divide the sweet potato brownies into 16 pieces and serve.

Nutrition: Calories 312 Fat 8 Fiber 5.9 Carbs 1.9 Protein 13

47.   Raspberry Brownies

Preparation Time: 50 minutes

Cooking Time 30 minutes

Servings: 4-6

Ingredients:

- `150 g dark chocolate
- `250 g butter
- `5 eggs
- `100 g raw cane sugar
- `1 tsp.. vanilla powder
- `180 g spelled flour type 630
- `3 tbsp.. cocoa powder
- `1 tsp.. baking powder
- `400 g raspberries

Directions:

1. Roughly chop the chocolate with a knife. Melt the butter with the chocolate over a hot water bath and then let it cool down slightly. Mix the eggs with the whole cane sugar and vanilla powder in a bowl until creamy white. Add the chocolate butter and stir in. Mix the flour with the cocoa and baking powder and stir into the chocolate mixture. Pour about half of the dough onto the baking sheet lined with baking paper (or in a baking pan) and spread it on top. Sprinkle the selected raspberries on top and smooth the rest of the batter over it.

2. Bake for about 15 – 20 minutes in a preheated oven (fan oven: 160 ° C; gas: level 2–3) to keep the pullover moist. Then pick it up and let it get cool. Cut into pieces and, if you like, serve powdered sugar.

Nutrition: Calories 222 Fat 2 Fiber 3.9 Carbs 2.3 Protein 17

48.   Brownie Cheesecake

Preparation Time: 50 minutes Cooking Time 30 minutes

Servings: 4-6

Ingredients:

- `100 g dark chocolate (70% cocoa content)
- `125 g room temperature butter
- `100 g raw cane sugar
- `3 eggs
- `300 g quark (20% fat)
- `125 g spelled flour type 1050
- `1/2 packet baking powder
- `1/2 tsp.. vanilla powder
- `1 pinch salt

Directions:

1. For the chocolate mass, roughly chop the chocolate over a hot, non-boiling water bath. Then let cool down a little.

2. Mix the butter with the raw cane sugar in a bowl until creamy. Stir in the eggs and quark. Mix the flour with baking powder, vanilla, and salt and stir the flour mixture into the batter. Divide the dough and stir in the chocolate under half.

3. Fill the baking tin alternately in 3–4 layers and carefully marble with a fork. Bake in a preheated oven at 180C for 30 minutes. Take out and let cool on a wire rack. Cut into pieces for serving.

Nutrition: Calories 387 Fat 5 Fiber 3 Carbs 3.9 Protein 11

49.   Zucchini-Brownies

Preparation Time: 30 minutes

Cooking Time 55 minutes

Servings: 6

Ingredients:

- `350 g zucchini
- `60 g coconut oil
- `50 g dark chocolate (70% cocoa content)
- `100 g whole meal spelled flour
- `100 g spelled flour (type 630)
- `80 g coconut blossom sugar
- `50 g cocoa powder
- `1 tsp.. baking powder
- `1/2 tsp.. vanilla powder
- `1 pinch salt
- `2 eggs

Directions:

1. Wash and grate the zucchini. Put in a sieve and squeeze out some liquid. Melt coconut oil in a small saucepan over low heat. Roughly chop the chocolate.

2. Put flours, coconut blossom sugar, cocoa powder, baking powder, vanilla powder, salt, eggs, and liquid coconut oil in a bowl. Process all ingredients with the whisk of a hand mixer to smooth dough. Mix in the zucchini well, fold in the chocolate.

3. Pour the dough into a pan lined with baking paper and smooth it out. Bake in a preheated oven at 180 C for 20–25 minutes (stick test). Then let cool completely in the mold. Cut into pieces and enjoy.

Nutrition: Calories 342 Fat 1 Fiber 8 Carbs 5 Protein 12

50. **Bean brownies**

Preparation Time: 30 minutes

Cooking Time 55 minutes

Servings: 6

Ingredients:

- `For the bean brownies
- `20th soft dates (soaked in hot water for 10 minutes)
- `180 g kidney beans (drained weight; can)
- `120 ml rapeseed oil
- `130 ml almond drink (almond milk) (or other vegetable milk)
- `3 eggs
- `50 g delicate oat flakes
- `50 g ground almond kernels
- `50 g cocoa powder
- `1 tsp.. baking powder
- `1 pinch salt
- `5 tbsp.. chopped walnut kernels
- `For the frosting
- `1 ripe avocado
- `3 tbsp.. coconut oil (melted)
- `3 tbsp.. espresso
- `3 tbsp.. cocoa powder
- `5 tbsp.. maple syrup
- `streusel or coarse sea salt as desired

Directions:

1. Puree the dates and kidney beans in a blender, food processor, or with a hand blender to a creamy purée.

2. Add rapeseed oil, almond drink, eggs, oat flakes, ground almonds, cocoa powder, baking powder, and salt to the date and bean puree and stir to make a brownie batter.

3. Fold the chopped walnuts into the dough and pour the dough into a baking dish (approx. 26 x 20 centimeters) lined with baking paper. Bake in a preheated oven at 180 C for about 30 minutes. Then let it cool down completely.

4. Now process all the ingredients for the frosting with a hand blender or a food processor into a fine chocolate cream and use a spatula to spread over the bean brownie. Refine with toppings as desired, cut into 16 pieces, and store in the refrigerator.

Nutrition: Calories 323 Fat 3 Fiber 3 Carbs 1.2 Protein 6

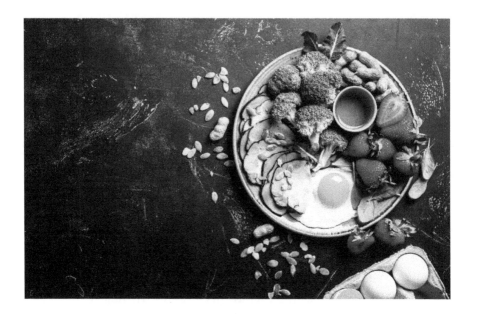

30 DAY MEAL PLAN

DAY	BREAKFAST	LUNCH	DINNER	DESSERTS
1	Egg Sausage Breakfast Casserole	Garlic Duck Breast	Pork Chops	Chocolate Mousse
2	Vegetable Omelet	Thyme Lamb Chops	Spicy Pork & Spinach Stew	Chocolate Chia Pudding With Almonds
3	Cheese Bacon Quiche	Autumn Pork Stew	Stuffed Taco Peppers	Coconut Macadamia Chia Pudding
4	Egg Breakfast Casserole	Handmade Sausage Stew	Chinese Pulled Pork	Keto Chocolate Mug
5	Cauliflower Breakfast Casserole	Marinated Beef Tenderloin	Bacon Wrapped Pork Loin	Vanilla Chia Pudding
6	Veggie Frittata	Chicken Liver Sauté	Lamb Barbacoa	Choco Lava Cake
7	Feta Spinach Quiche	Chicken In Bacon	Balsamic Pork Tenderloin	Coconut Cup Cakes
8	Cauliflower Mashed	Whole Chicken	Spicy Pork	Easy Chocolate Cheesecake
9	Kalua Pork With Cabbage	Duck Rolls	Zesty Garlic Pulled Pork	Chocolate Chip Brownie
10	Creamy Pork	Keto Adobo	Ranch	Coconut

	Chops	Chicken	Pork Chops	Cookies
11	Beef Taco Filling	Cayenne Pepper Drumsticks	Pork Chile Verde	Choco Pie
12	Flavorful Steak Fajitas	Keto Bbq Chicken Wings	Ham Soup	Keto Blueberry Muffins
13	Garlic Herb Pork	Sweet Corn Pilaf	Beef And Broccoli	Keto Oven-Baked Brie Cheese
14	Garlic Thyme Lamb Chops	Mediterranean Vegetable Mix	Korean Barbecue Beef	Keto Vanilla Pound Cake
15	Pork Tenderloin	Spaghetti Cottage Cheese Casserole	Garlic Chicken	Almond Roll With Pumpkin Cream Cheese Filling
16	Smoky Pork With Cabbage	Meatballs With Coconut Gravy	Lamb Shanks	No Bake Low Carb Lemon Strawberry Cheesecake
17	Italian Frittata	Fresh Dal	Jamaican Jerk Pork Roast	Pecan Cheesecake
18	Easy Mexican Chicken	Pulled Pork Salad	Salmon	Blueberry And Zucchini Muffins
19	Cherry Tomatoes Thyme	Garlic Pork Belly	Coconut Chicken	Coffee Mousse

	Asparagus Frittata			
20	Healthy Veggie Omelet	Sesame Seed Shrimp	Mahi Mahi Taco Wraps	Chocolate Cake
21	Scrambled Eggs With Smoked Salmon	Chicken Liver Pate	Shrimp Tacos	Sweet Potato Brownies
22	Persian Omelet Slow cooker	Cod Fillet In Coconut Flakes	Fish Curry	Raspberry Brownies
23	Keto Slow cooker Tasty Onions	Prawn Stew	Salmon With Creamy Lemon Sauce	Brownie Cheesecake
24	Crustless Slow cooker Spinach Quiche	Pork-Jalapeno Bowl	Salmon With Lemon-Caper Sauce	Zucchini-Brownies
25	Eggplant Pate With Breadcrumbs	Chicken Marsala	Spicy Barbecue Shrimp	Bean Brownies
26	Red Beans With The Sweet Peas	Chickpeas Soup	Lemon Dill Halibut	Luscious Walnut Chocolate Brownies
27	Nutritious Burrito Bowl	Hot And Delicious Soup	Coconut Cilantro Curry Shrimp	Gluten-Free Chocolate Cake
28	Quinoa Curry	Delicious	Shrimp In	Brownies

		Eggplant Salad	Marinara Sauce	With Nuts
29	Ham Pitta Pockets	Tasty Black Beans Soup	Garlic Shrimp	Halloween Brownies
30	Breakfast Meatloaf	Rich Sweet Potato Soup	Lemon Pepper Tilapia	Raw Brownies With Cashew Nuts

CONVERSION TABLES

Volume Equivalents (Liquid)

US STANDARD	US STANDARD (OUNCES)	METRIC (APPROXIMATE)
2 tablespoons	1 fl. oz...	30 mL
1/4 cup	2 fl. oz...	60 mL
1/2 cup	4 fl. oz...	120 mL
1 cup	8 fl. oz...	240 mL
11/2 cups	12 fl. oz...	355 mL
2 cups or 1 pint	16 fl. oz...	475 mL
4 cups or 1 quart	32 fl. oz...	1 L
1 gallon	128 fl. oz...	4 L

Volume Equivalents (Dry)

US STANDARD	METRIC (APPROXIMATE)
1/4 teaspoon	1 mL
1/2 teaspoon	2 mL
1 teaspoon	5 mL
1 tablespoon	15 mL
1/4 cup	59 mL
cup	79 mL
1/2 cup	118 mL
1 cup	177 mL

Oven Temperatures

FAHRENHEIT (F)	CELSIUS (C) (APPROXIMATE)
250°F	120 °C
300°F	150°C
325°F	165°C
350°F	180°C
375°F	190°C
400°F	200°C
425°F	220°C
450°F	230°C

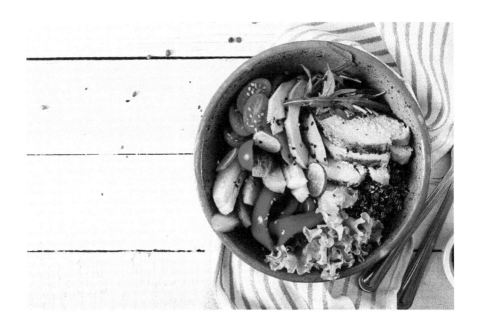

CONCLUSION

Now you can cook healthier meals for yourself, your family, and your friends that will get your metabolism running at the peak of perfection and will help you feel healthy, lose weight, and maintain a healthy balanced diet. A new diet isn't so bad when you have so many options from which to choose. You may miss your carbs, but with all these tasty recipes at your fingertips, you'll find them easily replaced with new favorites.

You will marvel at how much energy you have after sweating though the first week or so of almost no carbs. It can be a challenge, but you can do it! Pretty soon you won't miss those things that bogged down your metabolism as well as your thinking and made you tired and cranky. You will feel like you can rule the world and do anything, once your body is purged of heavy carbs and you start eating things that rejuvenate your body. It is worth the few detox symptoms when you actually start enjoying the food you are eating.

A Keto diet isn't one that you can keep going on and off. It will take your body some time to get adjusted and for ketosis to set in. This process could take anywhere between two to seven days. It is dependent on the level of activity, your body type and the food that you are eating.

There are various mobile applications that you can make use of for tracking your carbohydrate intake. There are paid and free applications as well. These apps will help you in keeping a track of your total carbohydrate and fiber intake. However, you won't be able to track your net carb intake. MyFitnessPal is one of the popular apps. You just need to open the app store on your smartphone, and you can select an app from the various apps that are available.

The amount of weight that you will lose will depend on you. If you add exercise to your daily routine, then the weight loss will be greater. If you cut down on foods that stall weight loss, then this will speed up the process. For instance, completely cutting out things like artificial sweeteners, dairy and wheat products and other related products will definitely help in speeding up your weight loss. During the first two weeks of the Keto diet, you will end up losing all the excess water weight. Ketosis has a diuretic effect on the body, and you might end up losing a couple of pounds within the first few days of this diet. After this, your body will adapt itself to burning fats for generating energy, instead of carbs.

You now have everything you need to break free from a dependence on highly processed foods, with all their dangerous additives that your body interprets as toxins. Today, when you want a sandwich for lunch, you'll roll the meat in Swiss cheese or a lettuce leaf and won't miss the bread at all, unless that is, you've made up the Keto bread recipe you discovered in this book! You can still enjoy your favorite pasta dishes, even taco salad, but without the grogginess in the afternoon that comes with all those unnecessary carbs.

So, energize your life and sustain a healthy body by applying what you've discovered. You don't have to change everything at once. Just start by adopting a new recipe each week that sounds interesting to you. Gradually, swap out less-than-healthy options for ingredients and recipes from this book that will promote your well-being.

Each time you make a healthy substitution or try a new ketogenic recipe, you can feel proud of yourself; you are actually taking good care of your mind and body. Even before you start to experience the benefits of a ketogenic lifestyle, you can feel good because you are choosing the best course for your life.

Thanks for reading.

Lightning Source UK Ltd.
Milton Keynes UK
UKHW020815020321
379644UK00001B/28